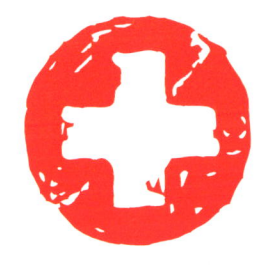

# The Traveler's Vest Pocket Medical Guide

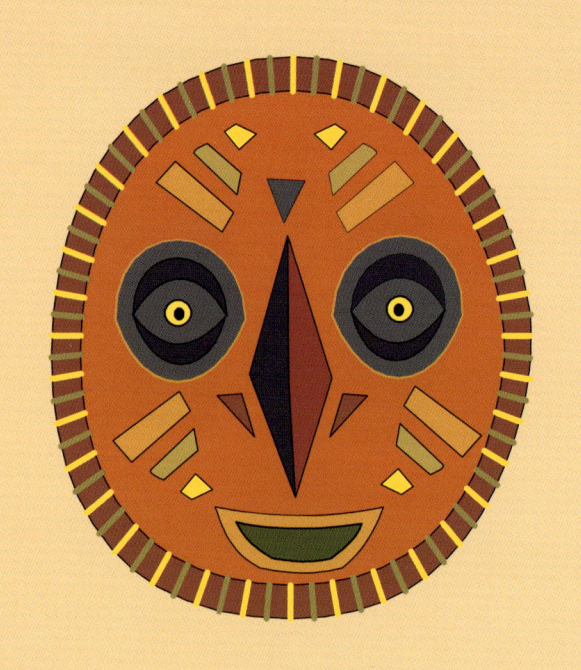

# The Traveler's Vest Pocket Medical Guide

*Identification and Treatment of Common Travel Maladies*

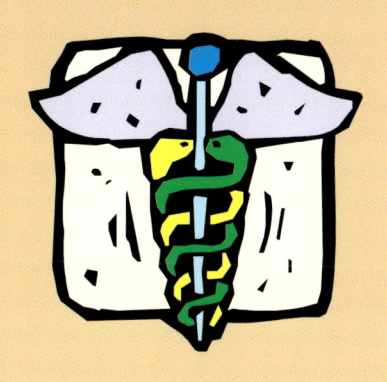

Morris Weiss, M.D.
W. Paul McKinney, M.D.

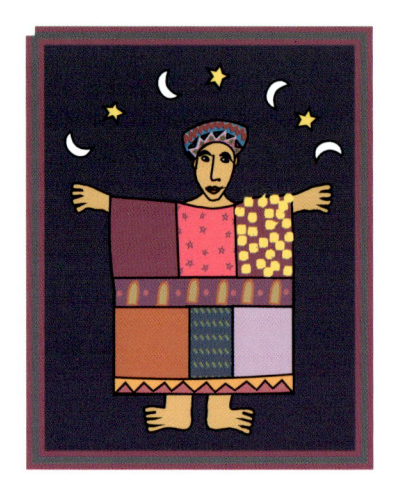

Copyright © 2000 by Dr. Morris Weiss
and Dr. W. Paul McKinney

All Rights Reserved.

ISBN 1-884532-37-3

Published by Butler Books
608 Briar Hill
Louisville, KY 40206
502-897-9393

No portion of this book may be reproduced by any mechanical,
digital or xerographic means without the prior written
permission of the copyright holders.

Printed in China

Dear Traveler;

Welcome to the only travel medical book you will ever need! It will help you prepare all your medical travel needs; deliver you in good condition to any exotic destination; and bring you home happy and healthy.

The tips found in this book will be especially useful for those of you who are adventure travelers, and who enjoy a bit of risk while seeing the world. This book may be the most important piece of equipment you'll carry. Read it and familiarize yourself with its sections *before* you leave; in an emergency you'll be much faster finding the information you need. As the Boy Scouts say, "Be prepared." This book gives you a full measure of preparedness.

Have a safe and happy trip.

Dr. Morris Weiss
Dr. W. Paul McKinney

## ABOUT THE AUTHORS

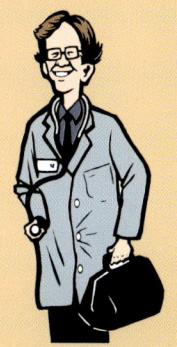

**Dr. Paul McKinney** is the V.V. Cooke Professor and Chief of the Division of General Internal Medicine at the University of Louisville Medical School. Dr. McKinney's research interests are in three areas: infectious disease epidemiology, prevention in primary care, and medical informatics. He maintains a strong interest in travel medicine, having developed software for use by health care professionals in counseling Americans traveling abroad. His ongoing interest in the field of infectious diseases and travel medicine is reflected in his joining the Center for Disease Control's Advisory Committee on Immunization Practices as a liaison member from the Association of Teachers of Preventive Medicine in June, 1998.

**Dr. Morris Weiss** is a practicing cardiologist with a keen interest in archaeology. At the age of 40 he began working at classical dig sites around the Mediterranean. Toiling away as a laborer at the excavation sites, he found that his medical knowledge was of value to team members who became ill or had difficulties adjusting to foreign travel and primitive living conditions. The combination of 35 years of medical practice and twenty years in the field has helped produce this book.

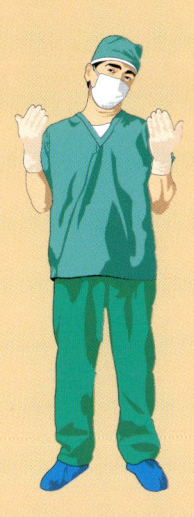

# TABLE OF CONTENTS

## SECTION ONE:
## What To Do Before You Leave

| | |
|---|---|
| A Basic Checklist of Travel Items and Pre-Trip Needs | *10-11* |
| A Basic Emergency Medicine Kit | *12* |
| A Basic First-Aid Kit | *13* |
| Other Necessities | *14-15* |

## SECTION TWO:
## What To Do On The Way

| | |
|---|---|
| Motion Sickness | *16* |
| Jet Lag | *17* |
| High Altitude Sickness | *17* |

## SECTION THREE:
## What To Do After You Arrive

| | |
|---|---|
| Water | *18-19* |
| Fluid intake | *20* |
| Personal Hygiene | *21* |
| Tips for Physical and Emotional Well-Being | *22* |
| What to Wear | *23* |
| Food | *24-25* |

# SECTION FOUR: THE TREATMENT GUIDE

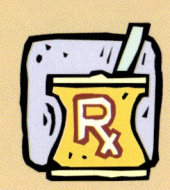

Rash, *29*

Fractures, *30*

Red Eye, *31*

Fungal Infections, *32*

Tick Bite, *33*

Jaundice, *34*

Ankle Injury, *35*

Chest Discomfort, *36-37*

Vomiting, *38-39*

Heart Palpitation, *40-41*

Animal Bites, *42-43*

Depression, *44*

Fish Hook, *45*

Constipation, *46*

Nose Bleed, *47*

Headache, *48*

Toothache, *49*

Earache, *50*

Bladder/Kidney Infection, *51*

Cuts, *52*

Head Injury, *53*

Abdominal Pain, *54-55*

Diarrhea, *56-57*

# Before You Leave

### Your Basic Checklist

Write down a list of the countries you wish to visit, then inquire from public health authorities (such as the Center for Disease Control—www.cdc.gov) about the basics regarding immunizations required for each of those countries; the need for specific medications for constant disease risk such as malaria; and special clothing needs.

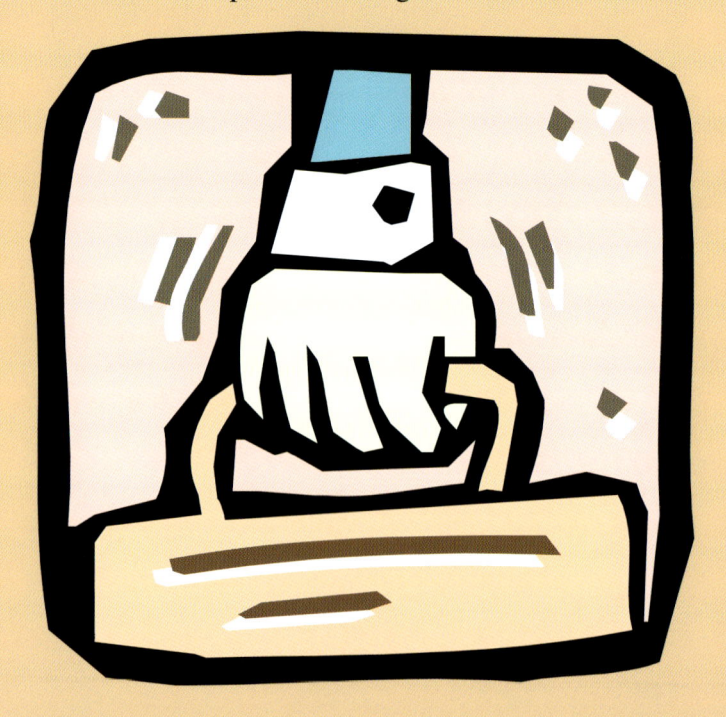

- Gather all the prescription or non-prescription medicines you take on a regular basis, and purchase a supply sufficient for the entire trip + two or three days. (You never know when your flights will be delayed.)

- List your allergies and blood type and put with your travel documents. Don't forget your medical insurance card.

- Visit your local travel medicine professional or your family doctor three months in advance of your departure date. If inoculations for your destination are needed, it's best to avoid getting them at the last minute. Otherwise it may mean traveling with a low grade fever, a sore arm or sore buttocks.

- If you have a chronic medical condition, be sure to consult your physician for an evaluation before you travel.

- Bring extra reading glasses and/or contact lenses, eye drops for contacts, and sunglasses.

- Put together your Basic First Aid Kit, your Emergency Medicine Kit, and your Necessities Kit (all found on the next four pages).

## YOUR BASIC EMERGENCY MEDICINE KIT

In addition to the medicines you take regularly, take along these basics (if they fit, put them in your First Aid Kit).

- **For Diarrhea**
    - Lomotil
    - or Imodium
- **For Motion or Air Sickness**
    - Dramamine (50 mg tablets)
- **For Headache or General Pain Relief**
    - Tylenol and/or Ibuprofen (Advil)
- **For heavy exertion in tropical/ subtropical climates**
    - salt tablets
- **For severe pain**
    - Tylenol with codeine
- **For allergic reactions**
    - Benadryl (50 mg)
- **Antibiotics**
    - Tetracycline (500 mg)
    - Amoxicillin (500 mg)
- **Antibiotic skin salve**
    - Bacitracin ointment or equivalent

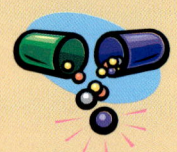

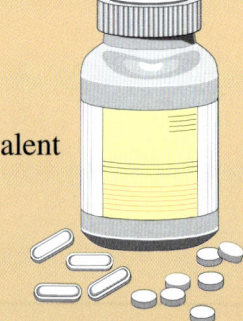

## YOUR BASIC FIRST AID KIT

You won't need a large travel bag or toiletries kit for these essentials, but get one that is big enough to hold it all comfortably, and, if possible, is waterproof.

- **Betadine (antiseptic)**
- **1-inch wide Band-aids**
- **Butterfly-type band-aids**
- **1-inch wide adhesive tape**
- **Elastic (Ace) bandage (best size is 3 inches wide)**
- **Sterile gauze pads**
- **Sterile gauze roll**
- **Sewing needle for splinters**
- **Small scissors**
- **Safety pins**
- **Tweezers**

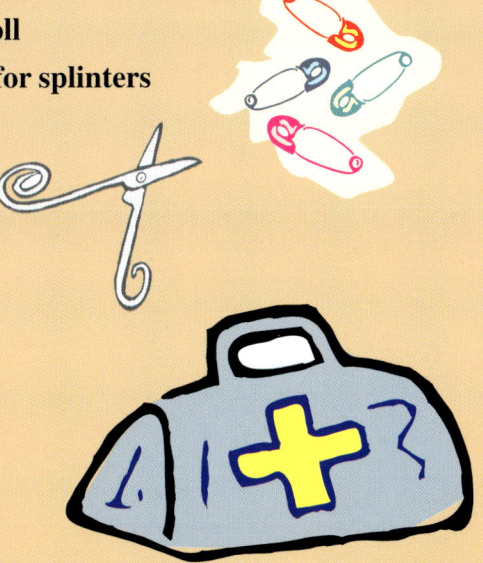

## OTHER NECESSITIES

Take these along, too, especially if you are going to remote locations.

- **Hand soap** (anti-microbial, e.g. Dial)

- **Tampons** (often hard to find overseas)

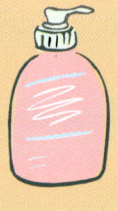

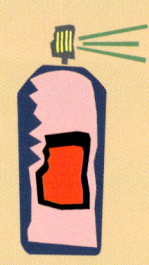

  - **Skin care items**
    - sunscreen in various SPFs
    - Bug repellant (no higher than 30% DEET)
    - "6/12"
    - "OFF"

  - **Calamine lotion** for itchy rashes

- **Talcum powder**
 (sprinkle on socks and underwear to prevent fungal infections)

- **Anti-fungal powders** (Miconazole to treat fungal infections)

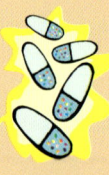

  - **Contraceptives** (Hard to find in the rain forest)

  - **Halazone** (Iodine) tablets to purify

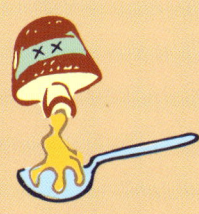

drinking water. When bottled or boiled water is not available, put two or more tablets in each quart of water, then wait 30 minutes for the full effect. Side effect: bad taste, but you'll get over it.

• **Laxative**

• **Antihistamines**/over-the-counter sinus medicine

• **Sunburn cream** (Noxzema)

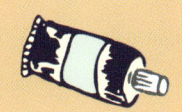

   • **Hemorrhoid preparation** (Anusol)

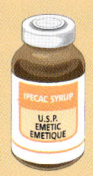

   • **Syrup of Ipecac** to induce vomiting in case of poisoning

   • **Antacids** (Mylanta, Rolaids, Tums)

• **Molefoam** for blisters

• **Pocket Knife**, especially a multi-purpose Swiss Army type

• **Thermometer** (digital if possible. If only a glass type is available, pack in a hard case).

**WARNING! Never pack glass containers. Use plastic at all times.**

# On the way...

1. For car, boat, train or airplane travel, make sure you have a **motion sickness medicine** within easy reach (not packed away in your suitcase):
    • Dramamine, or
    • Transderm Scop patch, or
    • Phenergan or Compazine

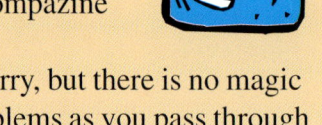

2. What about **jet lag**? Sorry, but there is no magic potion to avoid sleep problems as you pass through different time zones. Moving through three or more time zones usually causes some upset whether you are going east or west. Some "cures" purport to be out there, among them the controversial hormone, melatonin. The use of melatonin (according to its advocates) is complex regarding the best times of day to take it and whether one should be inside or outside under the sun. We remain skeptical about it, and all the other jet lag miracle cures. We find that if you drink plenty of fluids and attempt to sleep during your normal sleep hours, you will arrrive well rested. To know when it's time to sleep, you should keep your watch set to your "home time" during your outbound leg and change it only when you have adjusted to your new location. On the trip back, we suggest you sleep the first day according to the sleep

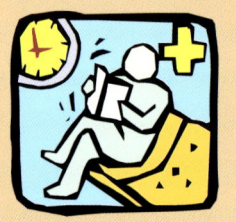

cycle you have adjusted to on your trip.

3. Many adventure destinations are located at high altitudes. To get there, you may be landing at a high altitude or will be climbing to a high altitude. If you know, or suspect, that you suffer from **high-altitude sickness**, and do not have two or three days to acclimate, start Diamox at 500 mg per day at least 24 hours before you leave, and continue taking it while you are at altitude.

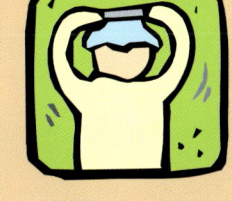

In addition to these drugs, we suggest you drink plenty of fluids, especially if you are landing at 10,000 feet (3,000 meters) or higher.

The most severe form of high altitude sickness produces acute pulmonary edema, in which the traveler experiences profound shortness of breath from fluid on the lungs. This problem usually occurs at 14,000 feet (4,242 meters) or above. The symptoms are alleviated only by moving down to 8,500 feet (2575 meters) as rapidly as possible.

## After You Arrive

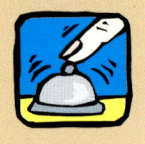

**ABOUT WATER!**
Our first bit of advice: **Consider all drinking water unsafe until proven otherwise.**

• In most of the world tap water is unsafe for both drinking and brushing teeth, but OK for bathing.

• Drink only bottled water. (You should personally uncap it.)

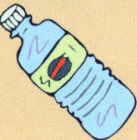

• Never drink soft drinks or beer unless you pop the cap personally or watch the waiter or your host do it.

• In a restaurant, drink only steaming hot tea or coffee. Avoid ice cubes except in the best restaurants in the most advanced countries.

• If you are in a rural area or are doing hard work where bottled water is unavailable, such as on an archaeological dig, we suggest the following:

1. Boil water for at least five minutes. At high altitudes, boil for a few minutes longer.

2. Carry a canteen with water purification tablets.

3. Wash dishes with soap and the safest possible local water; then thoroughly rinse all dishes, glasses, silverware, pots and pans with copious amounts of boiled water. Air dry the dishes, covering them with a mesh fabric of any material to protect them from flies. In rural villages where the animals live in the houses with the people, and dry dung is used as fuel for cooking and heating, hoards of flies are present. This is the norm in many parts of the world.

• If boiling water is impractical, use water purification tablets (Halazone). Dosage is two tablets per quart (liter) of water. Most personal canteens hold one quart of liquid.

• If you develop traveler's diarrhea, you must replace by mouth what you lose in the watery stool. Begin drinking immediately. Small sips will help avoid nausea and vomiting. In addition to water, hot tea, boiled broth and carbonated beverages are also helpful. These liquids replace valuable minerals and nutrients lost in the stool.

**And Don't Forget...**

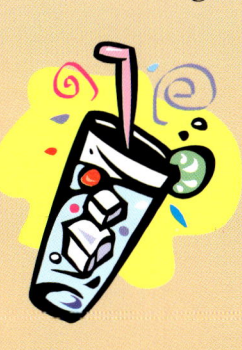

• Portable water filters are **not** to be trusted to eliminate the risk of infection.
• Adding alcohol to your drink does **not** purify the ice cubes or the water.
• Charcoal filtrating is ineffective
• Fresh fruit juices and milk are **not** to be drunk in most parts of the world.

- **Regarding fluid intake**:
The volume of fluid necessary per day for a person living in a temperate climate is 8 to 12 glasses, with each glass totaling 8 ounces (250 cc). Therefore you should be drinking between 2 and 3 quarts (2 and 3 liters) per day of either water, soup, soft drinks, tea, coffee, etc. For an active, perspiring individual, more fluid will be necessary. The best gauge of your need for fluids is the amount of urine that your body puts out in a 24-hour period. If you produce the equivalent of three 8-ounce glasses (750 cc's) of urine, your intake is just adequate.

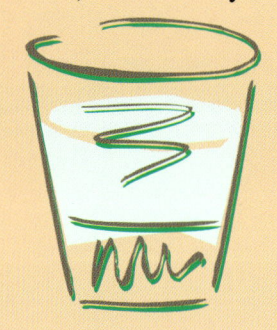

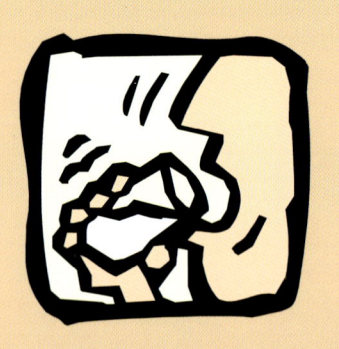

- In tropical or semi-tropical climates, you will need an extra 14 to 16 glasses of water each day. Often 4 to 6 salt tablets should be added to the water if heavy work or exercise is performed in hot, sunny weather. It's hard to drink too much liquid, and it is easy to not drink enough. If your urine volume begins to fall, drink more liquid. The amount of water needed in hot, dry climates is always more than you expect. So be prepared!

## PERSONAL HYGIENE

- Bathe daily with soap; check your skin and hair for ticks and other insect bites.

- Wash your hands with soap any time you go to the bathroom, and *always* before eating.

- Use only your own toothbrush, towel, hairbrush and comb. Do not borrow or lend these items.

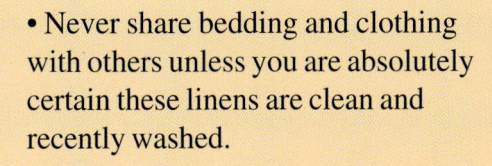

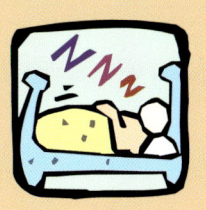

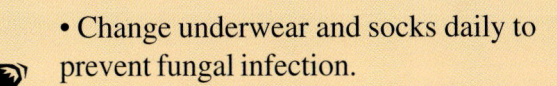

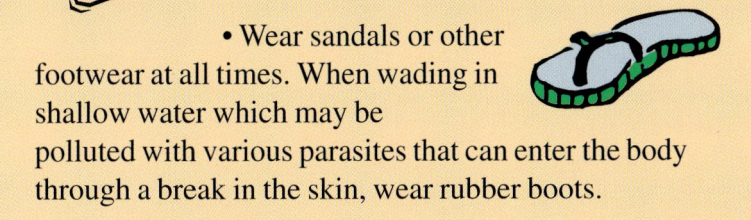

- Never share bedding and clothing with others unless you are absolutely certain these linens are clean and recently washed.

- Change underwear and socks daily to prevent fungal infection.

- Wear sandals or other footwear at all times. When wading in shallow water which may be polluted with various parasites that can enter the body through a break in the skin, wear rubber boots.

- Soak feet in chlorine solution before showering. This will help prevent athlete's foot. The solution should be available in any dorm or hostel setting.

• If an outside latrine is used, cover over each urination and bowel movement with lime.

• Sleep head to toe if in crowded dormitory, youth hostel or tent conditions.

**A Word About Local Medical Care:**
　　If you are trekking, working or living in a remote area of the world, there may be rural villages nearby. The likelihood of professional medical care there is near zero. Worse, if the villagers discover that you have medical supplies, then *you* may become the doctor. They might seek medical treatment. We find that in remote areas, people are almost mystical about western medicine. Of course, if there is a real medical emergency, you should try to help. As a rule, though, this is not a good idea. The line of people will soon be long, and if you don't treat them all, they will be upset!

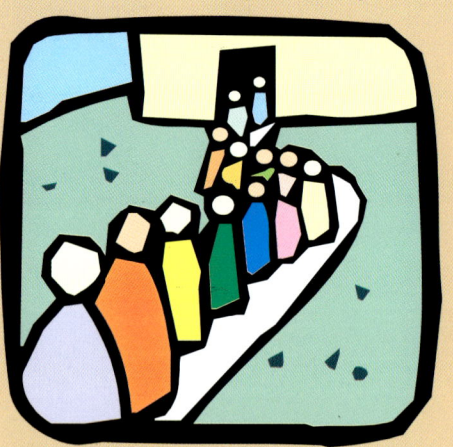

## TIPS FOR YOUR EMOTIONAL AND PHYSICAL WELL-BEING

• On your first trip abroad, you will probably try to do too much in too short a time. Why not give yourself a chance to get over your jet lag? We suggest that you go to bed earlier and sleep a bit later than usual in the morning, so that you will be fresh for whatever the day brings.

• Take a nap in the afternoon, especially in the siesta countries of the world. Follow the natives' example; avoid the heat of the day and relax after lunch.

• Loneliness and homesickness are common on a first trip overseas. We find that college students experience this on archaeology field trips or semesters of study abroad. The best thing to do is find someone to share your feelings with; if that's not possible, write letters home. Your sadness will soon pass.

• If teaching or missionary work bring you to an underdeveloped country, you may experience some initial disorientation. The initial frustration will dissipate once you learn a bit of the language, get used to the food, find a few friends, and understand the culture you've landed in. Be patient and your negative feelings will soon go away.

## WHAT TO WEAR

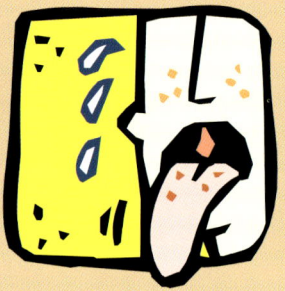

• Always have a hat. It's a must in the Mediterranean sun or in tropical or semi-trpical climates near the equator where the sun is intense.

• Wear loose cotton clothing in hot climates. Cotton is by far the coolest and most absorbent clothing fabric.

• Wear socks made of absorbent material, especially if lots of walking is on your agenda.

• Sunglasses are a requirement in tropical climates

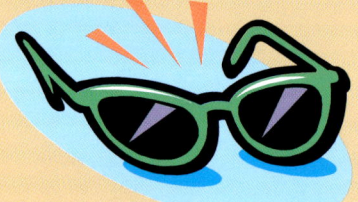

• In cold climates, we suggest you wear layers of loose-fitting clothing rather than one tight, heavy jacket. Layers trap body heat, and if you over-exert, you can always remove one or two layers.

• In cold climates wool fabrics are your best bet, along with new fabrics such as Polartek.

## FOOD IDEAS TO KEEP YOU HAPPY AND HEALTHY

First, a warning. Salads, raw vegetables, and peeled fresh fruit are to be considered table decorations (like cut flowers) unless you are in a three-star restaurant in Paris!

• When you buy fruits and vegetables, be certain that the skin is not broken. Scrub the food in drinking water with a mild detergent, then peel it yourself. Be sure to cook all vegetables. You can eat thick-skinned fruit raw only if you have cleaned and peeled it yourself. Never, never eat raw leafy vegetables; they cannot be cleaned thoroughly.

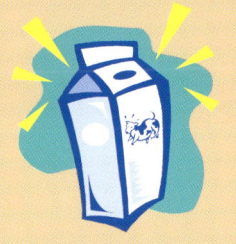

• Milk (except in advanced nations) is probably not pasteurized. If you have any doubts about its purity, boil it. Another idea is to mix dried milk powder with sterile water.

• Ice cream from street vendors is, in general, a bad idea. (The exception is Italy. They love their ice cream and it is always safe.)

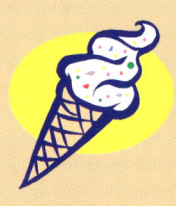

- Pastries, pies and custards, especially those with cream fillings, must come from a refrigerated source.

- Dry breads from most parts of the world can be considered safe.

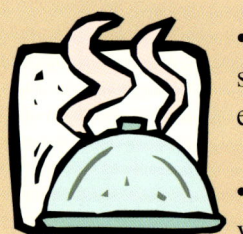

- All meats, eggs, fish, and shellfish must be cooked and eaten while still hot.

- It's not necessary to bring vitamins. Vitamin deficiencies take a long time to develop and rarely occur even under the most horrid dietary conditions.

- Remember that the body requires amazingly little protein to keep itself going. So if your travel duration is a few weeks or even months, enjoy the native fare even if it is low in protein. Just be sure that the food is well-cooked and hot.

- Unfamiliar spices could be a problem. If you need a little zing in your food, bring along your own spices from home. (There's always a Tabasco bottle around on a dig.)

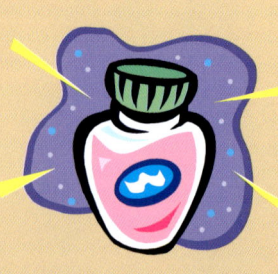

## A Few Other Caveats

• Olive oil is used in the Mediterranean area for cooking. For those unaccustomed to this food, diarrhea and abdominal pain from gallbladder upset may be common. You also may encounter these same symptoms from heavily fried foods found in the Middle East.

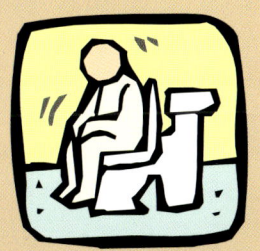

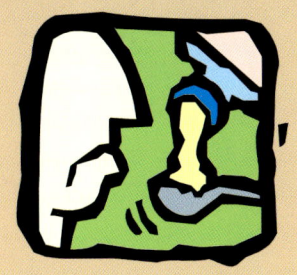

• Heartburn can occur after eating the heavily spiced foods in Central and South America, the Middle East, and the Indian subcontinent.

• If you are responsible for buying food for your group, remember that all meat and poultry must be freshly butchered. American-style refrigeration of foods is rare in many parts of the world.

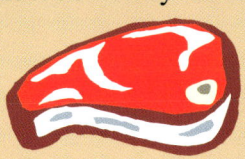

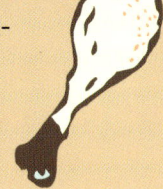

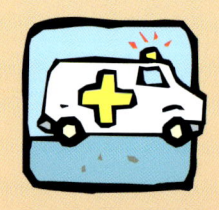

# THE TREATMENT GUIDE

This section is a guide to the treatment of many common medical problems the traveler encounters.

First look for your problem in the bold type at the top of the page, then follow the arrows to a rapid cure or course of treatment. These simple steps will guide you through the illness and relieve your anxiety about your condition. Rarely will you need to consult a physician. (The International Association for Medical Assistance to Travelers (IAMAT—see page 58) reference guide to English-speaking physicians located in most countries of the world can be obtained by calling 1-800-123-4567.)

NOTE: The information in this guide is completely accurate to the knowledge of the authors. It is intended to be used as a guide for medical care of common disorders while traveling. It is not intended to replace the advice of your own physician in case of a medical emergency. When in doubt, always consult a doctor.

# RASH

## No Fever

Discontinue all non-essential medications.

▼

If recently in the woods, consider poison ivy. For itching, use calamine lotion and benadryl.

## With Fever

Probably a sign of systemic infection (usually viral, such as measles).

▼

Use Tylenol (preferred). Use benadryl for itching. Observe for 24 hours. Encourage intake of fluids. **If situation worsens, see a doctor.**

▼

If insect bite preceded rash, **consult a physician before any treatment.**

# FRACTURES

**Simple**
(skin not broken)

Immobilize the bone with any available splint.

▼

Administer pain medication (Advil, Motrin).

▼

Transport for x-ray and cast.

**Compound**
(bone sticks out through the skin)

If bleeding, apply a tourniquet sufficiently tight to slow the bleeding.

▼

Immobilize and **transport immediately to a medical facility.**

▼

Administer pain medication. Lay injured person flat.

## RED EYE

For simple pain or slight redness, irrigate with sterile water or Visine. Check eye for dust or particles. Most symptoms will disappear within a few hours. Wear sunglasses for light sensitivity.

▼

If pain worsens or drainage from the eye develops, **seek medical attention.**

If there is pronounced sensitivity to light, or loss of vision, do not wait—**see a doctor immediately**.

# FUNGAL INFECTIONS

Most commonly, athlete's foot or jock itch.

▼

Treat locally as soon as possible with Clotrimazole (Lotrimin) or Miconazole (Micatin). Use Desenex only for athlete's foot.

▼

Keep socks, shoes and underwear dry and clean. Change socks and underwear daily. Keep feet and groin clean and dry. Bathe daily.

## TICK BITE

### Tick unattached

Wash the area and apply disinfectant.

▼

Note tick coloration, markings and date of bite. **If symptoms develop, contact physician and relate those details.** Symptoms often include rash, fever and muscle aches.

### Tick attached

Remove with constant, gentle pressure, using tweezers and tissue covering the fingers. After it is removed, wash the area and apply disinfectant.

▼

Note tick coloration and markings and date of bite. **If symptoms develop, contact physician and relate those details.** Symptoms often include rash, fever and muscle aches.

# JAUNDICE

### Yellow eyes and/or skin

When symptoms of yellowness of eyes or skin are obvious:

▼

**Seek medical attention immediately.**

▼

There are many possible causes, all of which require the attention of a physician and further testing and evaluation.

## ANKLE INJURY

### Pain but no swelling

Probably a strain.

▼

Rest the ankle, elevate it as much as possible.

▼

Apply ice (30 min.)

▼

Wrap with an Ace bandage.

▼

Tape it if walking is necessary.

### Pain with swelling

*If ankle not deformed:*

Rest the ankle; elevate it; ice it for 30 minutes; tape it if necessary.

*If ankle is deformed:*

Probably a fracture; do not put any weight on it; **seek a doctor's help.**

▼

Elevate it, ice it; take a pain reliever.

▼

Splint if possible.

## CHEST PAIN/DISCOMFORT

### *Mild Symptoms:*

- Sharp pain with or without deep breathing, lasting seconds to hours.
- Pain changes with body position
- Relief from belching or common antacids (Tums)

▼

### *Action:*

- Wait it out. Not likely to be a heart problem
- Eat lighter.
- Ibuprofen (Advil, Motrin) or Tylenol for pain with movement.
- Antacids for gas pressure.

## CHEST PAIN/DISCOMFORT

*<u>Moderate Symptoms:</u>*

•Noticeable chest pressure after exertion that melts away in 3-10 minutes with rest.

▼

•May be heart-related.
•**Avoid excessive exertion until you can consult a doctor**, especially if you are over 50.

*<u>Severe Symptoms</u>*

•Severe chest pain, possibly spreading to arms, neck or jaw.
•Sweating.
•Shortness of breath.

▼

•**Go to the nearest hospital, especially if over 50, to rule out heart attack.**

# VOMITING

### *Vomiting alone or with diarrhea and little-to- no belly pain:*

Probably food poisoning or viral origin.

Stop intake of solid foods.

▼

Keep up fluid intake with sips of tea, bottled water; soft drinks; mineral drinks (Gatorade).

▼

Phenergan or similar medication for persistent nausea.

▼

Imodium or Lomotil for diarrhea.

▼

**Seek medical help if no relief in 8 to 12 hours, and if urination stops.**

## VOMITING

***Vomiting with severe belly pain:***

**Seek medical help from the onset of the illness.**

***Bloody Vomiting***
***(Bright red or black):***

**Rush to the nearest hospital.**

## PALPITATION (IRREGULAR and/or FAST HEART BEAT AND PULSE)

### *Fast and Regular Pulse*

**Pulse between 100-150 per min. at neck or wrist**

Take fluids if thirsty.

▼

Tylenol preferred for fever.

▼

Lie down if dizzy.

▼

**See a doctor if fainting occurs** or no improvement in 24 hours.

**Pulse over 150/min.**

Sit or lie down if feeling faint.

▼

Gently gag to see if pulse slows.

▼

Take fluids if dehydrated.

▼

**See a doctor if there is chest pain,** shortness of breath, or symptoms last longer than a few hours, especially if over 60.

## PALPITATION (IRREGULAR and/or FAST HEART BEAT AND PULSE)

*Irregular Pulse*

**Pulse under 100/min.**

Try to relax. This is rarely dangerous.

▼

Eliminate caffeine and stimulant medicines from diet.

▼

Symptoms can be more prominent at night than when active.

**Pulse over 100/min.**

Take rest and fluids.

▼

**See doctor immediately** for chest pain, shortness of breath, dizziness, or if there is a history of heart disease.

▼

If symptoms last more than 12 hours, see a doctor.

# ANIMAL BITES/SCRATCHES

### *Bites/scratches with no break in skin*

Animal saliva may cause contamination through pre-existing breaks in skin, or through eye exposure.

### *Bites/scratches causing break in skin*

Tetanus shots up to date? Immediately clean wound using soap, lots of warm water and disinfectant.

▼

Is country rabies free? See list on next page

▼

If no, was animal captured?

▼

If yes, contact authorities to quarantine or sacrifice animal to obtain rabies test.
**If no, seek medical care immediately.**

## HIGH RISK ANIMALS FOR RABIES:
•Dogs•Bats•Raccoons•Foxes•Wolves

## ANIMALS NEVER RABID:
•Birds•Rodents•Reptiles

## COUNTRIES FREE OF RABIES

| Region | Country |
| --- | --- |
| Americas | Bermuda, St. Pierre and Miquelon |
| Caribbean | Anguilla, Antigua and Barbuda, Bahamas, Barbados, Cayman Islands, Dominica, Guadeloupe, Jamaica, Martinique, Montserrat, Netherlands Antilles (Aruba, Bonaire, Curacao, Saba, St. Maarten and St. Eustatius), St. Christopher (St. Kitts) and Nevis, St. Lucia, St. Martin, St. Vincent and Grenadines, Turks and Caicos Islands, Virgin Islands (U.K. and U.S.) |
| Asia | Bahrain, Hong Kong, Japan, Kuwait, Malaysia, Maldives, Singapore, Taiwan |
| Europe | Cyprus, Denmark, Faroe Islands, Finland, Gibraltar, Greece, Iceland, Ireland, Malta, Monaco, Norway (mainland), Portugal, Spain (except Ceuta/Melilla), Sweden, United Kingdom (Britain and Northern Ireland) |
| Pacific Oceana | Virt. all major and minor islands free of rabies |

## COUNTRIES *NOT* FREE OF RABIES

| | |
| --- | --- |
| Africa | No country absolutely free of rabies. |
| So. America | No country absolutely free of rabies. |

# DEPRESSION

### *Common mild symptoms:*

Crying.
Loss of appetite.
Insomnia.

▼

What to do:
- Be a good listener.
- Empathy is important.
- Keep person busy and active.

### *Rare, severe symptoms:*

Hallucinations.
Bizarre behavior.
Threatening suicide.

▼

What to do:
**Seek medical help immediately.**

# FISH HOOK IN SKIN

Push hook through skin with barb forward.

▼

Cut off barb point with wire cutter.

▼

Pull out remainder of hook.

**Note: If in or near the eye, go directly to a doctor or hospital.**

# CONSTIPATION

### *History:*

• No bowel movement for 2-5 days (Common with overseas travel).
• Gaseous and bloated at times.
Note: Constipation does not cause vomiting or blood in the stool.

### *What to do:*

Don't worry. No one dies of constipation. Be patient; it will happen.

▼

Drink plenty of bottled water.

▼

After 4 days if worried or uncomfortable, take a laxative. Look for magnesium citrates or phenolphthalein. Avoid irritants like castor oil.

▼

If abdomen becomes swollen or painful, **seek a doctor's help** (See page 54 for Abdominal Pain).

## NOSE BLEED

Don't panic; the bleeding will stop.

▼

Squeeze soft part of nose between thumb and forefinger.

▼

Ice on the bridge of the nose can help.

▼

Try not to swallow blood.

▼

**If it will not stop, go to emergency room for a nose pack.**

# HEADACHE

### *No fever:*
Tylenol or Ibuprofen (Advil)

### *Fever over 100.5 degrees*

*Symptoms:*
- Diarhhea
- Cough
- Body ache

**What to do:**

Take fluids by mouth

▼

Rest as much as possible

▼

Take pain reliever

▼

Take Imodium or Lomotil for diarrhea

*Symptoms:*
- Vomiting
- Stiff neck
- Pain with neck movement
- Confusion

**What to do:**

**Seek immediate medical advice.**

## TOOTHACHE

### *Pain only*

Take pain medication until you can see a dentist.

▼

Little risk of serious illness.

### *Pain, swollen jaw, fever and/or pus draining from tooth*

Seek dental care immediately

▼

Probably will need an antibiotic or a tooth extraction.

# EARACHE

## *Pain only*

*1. Cause: High altitude*
**What to do:**

Yawn or swallow frequently

▼

Close mouth, hold nose and try to blow nose

*2. Cause: Allergy history or mild cold*
**What to do:**

Tylenol or Advil

▼

Antihistamine

▼

Vaporizer at night.

## *Pain, fever, discharge from ear canal*

**What to do:**

**See a doctor**. May take simple pain medication and pseudoephedrine (Sudafed).

## BLADDER/KIDNEY INFECTION

(Burning sensation on urination
and/or frequency of urination)

### *No fever; no back or flank pain*

Drink plenty of liquids

▼

**See a doctor** if symptoms last more than 24 hours

### *Fever over 100.5 degrees and/or back/flank pain*

Drink plenty of fluids

▼

If over age 18 and not pregnant, take the Ciprofloxacin from your Basic Emergency Medical Kit.

▼

**See a doctor for antibiotics** if no improvement in 36 hours.

## CUTS

Irrigate with water and the Betadine in your Basic First Aid Kit; repeat.

▼

Apply pressure to control bleeding.

▼

Apply bandage from Basic First Aid Kit.

▼

For finger cut: If unable to bend normally, see a physician to determine if tendon is cut.

## HEAD INJURY

### *Unconscious*

**See a doctor immediately.**

### *Conscious*

Observe carefully before seeing a doctor.

▼

Take measures to prevent a second head trauma.

▼

**See a doctor immediately** if any of these symptoms occur:
- double vision
- obvious pupil dilation
- vomiting
- confusion
- memory loss
- stumbling, lack of balance

## ABDOMINAL PAIN

Mild abdominal pain is commonly present with diarhhea, with or without vomiting.

▼

*If blood is present*

**See a doctor immediately** if abdominal pain is accompanied by:
- blood in the urine
- blood with vomiting
- blood with bowel movements
- *For women*: blood from non-menstrual vaginal bleeding

**(Abdominal Pain, cont.)**

*If blood is not present*

**See a doctor immediately:**

- If pain is specifically in the lower right part of the abdomen

- If pain is accompanied by a rigid, board-like abdominal wall

- If pain is worsened by simple movement like riding in a car

- If there is an inability to consume or keep down liquids for a prolonged period

- If jaundice is present (yellowing of skin and eyes)

- If there is a high fever, but no diarrhea

- If pain is of great severity

## DIARRHEA

*For adults (over age 18)*

Take Ciprofloxacin (500 mg) by mouth twice daily (if not pregnant).

▼

Add Lomotil or Imodium at the onset for relief of cramps and frequent bowel movements. (Do not use for longer than 48 hours. Do not use if fever is higher than 102 degrees or if there is blood in the stool.

▼

Replace liquids lost in watery stool with liquids by mouth (sips). For rehydration, consider use of World Health Organization-recommended Oral Rehydration Salts (ORS) Solution, available at stores and pharmacies in most developing countries. Add one packet to boiled or treated water.

▼

**See a doctor** for any of the following:
- Persistence beyond 3 days
- Shaking chills
- Inability to keep down fluids

**(Diarrhea, cont.)**

*For children*

Do not use Ciprofloxacin. There are no generally recommended antibiotics for traveler's diarrhea in children.

May use Lomotil or Imodium if over 2 years old

Concentrate on rehydration. Oral Rehydration Salts solution is preferred (see previous page).

**See a doctor** if child
- Is unable to produce urine for several hours
- Is sleepy and not easily roused
- has sunken eyes
- has persistent vomiting

## IAMAT: The International Association for Medical Assistance to Travelers

One of the most worrisome problems for international travelers is how to deal with illness or other health emergencies in a foreign country. The traveler is under psychological and physical stress and often he has not only to cope with foreign languages and customs but with different food, water, climate, altitude and environmental hazards. There is a good chance, too, that the traveler's own immunities do not match the foreign local environment.

How can you learn about health risks in the different countries, the immunizations you need for your protection and where to turn if a medical problem arises?

You can become a member of IAMAT. A non-profit Foundation established in 1960, the aim of the organization is to advise travelers of health risks, geographical distribution of diseases, immunization requirements for all countries, and to make competent medical care available to the traveler around the world by doctors who speak either English or French besides their mother tongue and who had medical training in a western country.

For your personal membership card and package of IAMAT publications, contact one of the IAMAT membership offices listed below. Pleae be sure to include your complete mailing address.

**U.S.A.**
417 Center Street
Lewiston, NY 14092
TEL: (716) 754-4883
iamat@sentex.net

**Canada**
40 Regal Road,
Guelph, Ontario
N1K 1B5
TEL: (519) 836-0102
FAX: (519) 836-3412
E-MAIL: iamat@sentex.net

**New Zealand**
P.O. Box 5049
Christchurch 5
FAX: (643) 352-4630
E-MAIL: iamat@chch.planet.org.nz

**Switzerland**
57 Voirets
1212 Grand-Lancy-Geneva
(For written requests only)

As well as the many free publications IAMAT offers to its members, the items listed below are available at a nominal charge.

## IAMAT World Climate Charts

IAMAT publishes a series of 24 charts, each covering 60 cities, with detailed information about the sanitary conditions of water, milk and food, the monthly average maximum and minimum temperatures, the average rate of humidity and rainy days per month, and includes suggestions for clothing to be worn. These charts come in complete sets of 24 only, and a donation for these charts is requested as this is our fundraising project.

## LaMosquette™ Mosquito Beds

IAMAT also produces a portable, free-standing mosquito bed net of classical rectangular design. It is roomy and lets you sit up in bed without touching the netting. The net's holes are small enough to prevent the smallest mosquito from entering but large enough to allow for good airflow. This is of great importance for the humid and hot climates of malarious areas.

      LaMosquette is not only an important weapon against malaria, but will also protect against spiders, ticks, beetles, flies, roaches, assassin bugs, bed bugs and other insects. The net is sold at cost at our membership offices.

      Cost: US $110 plus postage.